Mangosteen

A Healthy Taste of the Tropics

Fruits of Paradise

Barbara Wexler, MPH

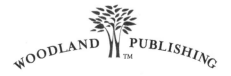

For permissions, ordering information, or bulk quantity discounts, contact: Woodland Publishing, 448 East 800 North, Orem, Utah 84097

Visit our Web site: www.woodlandpublishing.com
Toll-free number: (800) 777-2665

The information in this book is for educational purposes only and is not recommended as a means of diagnosing or treating an illness. All matters concerning physical and mental health should be supervised by a health practitioner knowledgeable in treating that particular condition. Neither the publisher nor the author directly or indirectly dispenses medical advice, nor do they prescribe any remedies or assume any responsibility for those who choose to treat themselves.

Cataloging-in-Publication data is available from the Library of Congress.

ISBN-13: 978-1-58054-470-2
ISBN-10: 1-58054-470-3

Printed in the United States of America

07 08 09 10 1 2 3 4 5 6 7 8 9 10

Contents

Fruits of Paradise Series

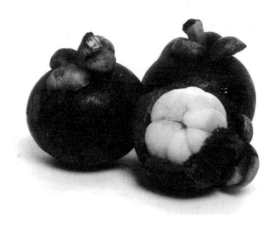

The Most Delicious Fruit in the World

Chances are good that you've never heard of, or even seen, a mangosteen. If you've guessed that it's an exotic tropical fruit, like its more familiar and similarly named distant kin, the mango, then you are correct. But a mangosteen (*Garcinia mangostana* L.) looks nothing like a mango and is not related to it, other than the fact that both are fruits. Mangosteen is a small round fruit—about two to three inches in diameter—the size of a peach, plum, or nectarine, with a thick, brittle, deep purple spherical outer shell. Its shell must be twisted and broken apart or cut with a knife to reveal the segmented bright white fruit nestled in the dark red outer pod. The number of fruit pods is the same as the number of bright green waxy petals on the bottom of the shell.

The average mangosteen shell holds four to eight fruit pods and the indescribably delicious edible snow white fruit may be seeded or seedless. The choicest fruits are those with the highest number of lobes at the top, because they have the highest number of fleshy segments and the fewest seeds.

Prized among fruits in Thailand, mangosteen is called the "queen of fruits," in contrast to the durian—a large Southeast Asian fruit with a creamy, gelatinous texture and pungent aroma and flavor that many Americans find distasteful—which is known as the "king of fruits." In contrast, the mangosteen is small, moist, and delicate; the juicy fruit pulp of the mangosteen is sweet and tangy with a scent that many people compare to strawberries, grapes, peaches, apples, pineapples, lychee, kiwi, plums, and papaya. The succulent flesh, divided into sections like an orange, almost melts in your mouth. Many people describe mangosteen as the most delicious fruit in the world.

If you've never seen a mangosteen, you're not alone. Very few people in the continental United States know the fresh fruit because, although it is grown on some of the islands of Hawaii, it is rarely exported to the mainland because of fears that the imported fruit might inadvertently transport Asian fruit flies into the United States where they could harm U.S. crops. The law requires that the fresh whole fruit that enters the United States be fumigated to ensure that it does not harbor fruit flies.

But if you're a devotee of Asian grocery stores then you may have spied fresh mangosteen, or at least frozen or canned mangosteen. It's also available as preserves, dried fruit, syrup, and a purplish jelly made from the rind and juice that many people describe as "ambrosia." When the seeds are included in processing the fruit, they add a subtle nutty flavor to mangosteen products.

The fresh fruit is generally eaten as a dessert, and the preserves or syrup as a topping for ice cream or sherbet. Although it is celebrated for its delicate, sweet, tart flavor, the fruit also has a long history of medicinal use in China and in ayurvedic medicine. Traditional Chinese medicine considers durian, a yang or hot food, while mangosteen is thought to have cooling, yin properties.

Traditional Medicinal Uses of Mangosteen

For centuries, people in Southeast Asia have used dried mangosteen rind, called pericarp, for medicinal purposes. Unripe mangosteen pericarp is about a half-centimeter thick and green; it darkens to purple when the fruit ripens. In China, it is powdered and given to people suffering from dysentery. A portion of the rind is steeped in water overnight and adults and children take the infusion as a remedy for chronic diarrhea. Along with its use to relieve symptoms of inflammatory bowel diseases and other gastrointestinal problems, mangosteen has been employed as an antiseptic, anti-inflammatory, antiparasitic, and antipyretic (an agent that prevents or reduces fever) as well as a pain and headache reliever. It also has been used to treat infections and skin rashes, and to soothe burns.

The Chinese and Thais rely on the antimicrobial and antiseptic actions of mangosteen to treat infected wounds, tuberculosis, malaria, urinary tract infections, and sexually transmitted diseases. The rind is boiled in water to extract its active ingredients and administered to relieve cystitis (inflammation of the bladder, usually caused by a bacterial infection) and gonorrhea. It is compounded into an ointment used to relieve eczema and other skin disorders and is applied to the skin as an astringent lotion.

In the Philippines, mangosteen leaves and bark are boiled and the resulting extract is used to reduce fever and to treat thrush (a potentially serious fungal infection of the throat and mouth), diarrhea, dysentery, and urinary tract disorders. In Malaya, an infusion of the leaves, combined with unripe banana and a little benzoin (balsamic resin of the Benjamin tree) is applied topically to ease the pain of circumcision. A distillate of boiled mangosteen root—a kind of mangosteen tea—is used to regulate menstruation, and a bark extract called amibiasine, has been used as an antiparasitic to treat amoebic dysentery. In the Caribbean, a tea made from mangosteen is used as a tonic for fatigue and malaise, and Brazilians use a similar brew as a deworming agent and to enhance digestion.

Modern Medicinal Uses of Mangosteen

In recent years, health-care practitioners have explored the use of mangosteen to:

- Relieve symptoms associated with arthritis and other musculoskeletal and joint problems
- Treat a variety of skin conditions including eczema, psoriasis, and seborrhea
- Help people with diabetes control their blood sugar levels
- Treat bacterial, fungal, and viral infections
- Help to heal ulcers in the mouth
- Relieve symptoms of asthma and allergies
- Prevent atherosclerosis—clogging, narrowing, and hardening

of the large arteries and medium-sized blood vessels, which can lead to stroke, heart attack, kidney disease, and eye problems
- Reduce mild to moderate anxiety and depression
- Relieve symptoms associated with gastric and duodenal ulcers, irritable bowel syndrome, ulcerative colitis, Crohn's disease, and diverticulitis
- Treat sleep disorders
- Provide antioxidant protection against free radicals

Today, pioneering researchers are investigating the potential of mangosteen extracts as adjuvant therapy (therapy that complements rather than replaces conventional treatment) for cancer patients, to prevent and treat cardiovascular disease, and to boost the immune system.

The Active Ingredients in Mangosteen

Mangosteen contains a class of compounds called xanthones, including alpha-mangostin, beta-mangostin, gamma-mangostin, garcinone B, and garcinone E, along with mangostinone, tannins, and a flavonoid called epicatechin. The rind of partially ripe fruits contains a polyhydroxy-xanthone derivative termed mangostin, or ß-mangostin. The rind of fully ripe fruits contains the xanthones. Mangosteen pulp also contains vitamins and minerals, including calcium, phosphorus, iron, thiamin, riboflavin, niacin, and ascorbic acid.

Xanthones are colorless crystalline compounds that occur naturally in various organic compounds. Xanthones have been derived from salicylate and used in the manufacture of some yellow dyes and insecticides. The xanthones that occur in nature, such as those derived from the mangosteen, are extracted from the rind or pericarp.

Xanthones are considered to have antioxidant properties that help to protect the body from the harm associated with free radicals. The human body routinely produces free radicals and these unstable chemicals are highly reactive and can oxidize other molecules very quickly. Once formed, free radicals can start a chain reaction of cell damage that ultimately results in the death of the cell.

Tannins are astringent, complex aromatic compounds found in the vacuoles (fluid-filled bubbles inside the cell) of certain plant cells. They are present in bark, leaves, and unripe fruit. Tannins produce a sensation as opposed to a taste or smell. The sensation is sometimes compared to over-steeped tea—it leaves your mouth feeling dry, with a slightly bitter taste, depending on how it hits the back of your tongue, where you taste bitterness. Tannins are responsible for the astringent flavor of unripe fruit and many red wines.

Tannins are naturally occurring plant polyphenols (antioxidant compounds) that bind and precipitate proteins. Some are glucosides, glycosides derived from glucose that are common in plants and rare in animals. These glucosides are thought to confer protection to the plant or to contribute to pigment formation since they are orange, yellow, and amber. They are strongly astringent and are used in tanning and dyeing. In fruit, tannins slow oxidation and act as natural preservatives. In medicine, tannins are used in antidiarrheal, hemostatic (agents to stop bleeding), and antihemorrhoidal compounds. Epicatechin is an important bioflavonoid. Bioflavonoids are also called flavonoids and are best known for their antioxidant activity. Bioflavonoids have been termed "natural biological response modifiers" because of their ability to adapt and moderate the body's reaction to microbes—allergens, viruses, and carcinogens (cancer-causing agents). They have demonstrated antiallergenic, anti-inflammatory, antimicrobial, and anticancer activity. Bioflavonoids also serve as powerful antioxidants, protecting against oxidative and free-radical damage. Epicatechin improves dilation of blood vessels, circulation, and blood flow, and for this reason has been used to support heart health.

The Importance of Antioxidants

We've all heard that nutrients called antioxidants are important to our health. But if we look closely at the word *antioxidant* it seems like a paradox. After all, oxygen is essential to our well-being. Why should we want to oppose it with an antioxidant? Breathing oxygen connects us to life. If the brain is deprived of oxygen for more than a few minutes, irreparable damage occurs, followed by death. So why should the body need an abundance of antioxidants—chemicals that fight the effects of oxygen?

The answer to this question lies in the subtle distinction between oxygenation and oxidation, a truly profound difference that takes us back to the evolutionary roots of the one hundred trillion cells in our bodies. The two-faced nature of oxygen—on the one hand an essential nutrient that we can't live without, and on the other a savage destroyer that must be blocked and opposed—is known as the oxygen paradox.

The oxygen paradox

The human body thrives in the presence of oxygen. Our cells burn sugars and fats in the presence of oxygen through an incredibly efficient aerobic (oxygen utilizing) biochemical process called the Krebs cycle (also called the citric acid cycle or the tricarboxylic acid cycle [TCA]). This constructive use of oxygen to generate cellular energy is called oxygenation. As long as oxygen is carefully directed into aerobic biochemical processes like the Krebs cycle, it's truly man's best friend.

The diagram below provides a glimpse into the complexity of the Krebs cycle, which in turn, is just a small part of the network of chemical reactions that make up our human metabolism and internal biological terrain.

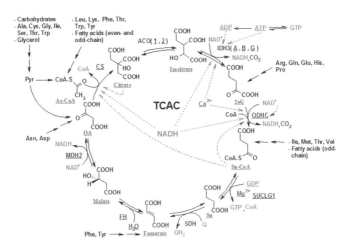

But oxygen has another face, we see every day whenever we look at metallic objects that have been left out in the elements to weather and rust. Oxygen is a highly reactive, corrosive chemical. It can turn the strongest iron chain into a weak and crumbling wreck by corrupting it, one atom at a time, through a process known as oxidation.

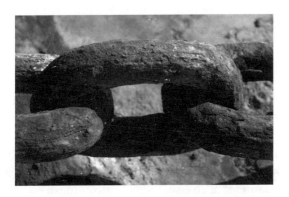

Oxidation is a process in which oxygen (or certain other chemicals) attach themselves to other substances by stripping away their electrons. In the case of rust, oxygen attaches to iron to form oxide compounds that weaken and corrode the original structure.

Inside the living body, something very similar can take place. Oxygen is capable of stripping an electron from another biochemical compound—effectively changing it into a positively charged ion since it has given up a negatively charged electron.

Sometimes this positive ion attaches to the oxygen or another negatively charged material. But on other occasions, the positively charged ion—which is now hungry for an electron so it can get back into electrical balance—strips an electron from a neighboring molecule, balancing itself but creating a new, imbalanced ion. The newly stripped ion can repeat this process and, like a line of dominos falling over, each one knocking down the next, a long chain of chemical changes can take place, each one damaging and degrading a previously balanced and functional biochemical substance.

Staying between the lines

As long as the oxygen within our bodies is directed into aerobic processes like the Krebs cycle, everything works perfectly. It's like cars speeding down the highway at sixty miles an hour. As long as they stay in their lanes, traffic flows along nicely and everyone travels smoothly and safely. But if the system of lanes breaks down and cars start weaving and moving around in every possible direction, then the situation immediately becomes dangerous and inefficient. It's the same way with oxygen, except that instead of painted lines to mark off lanes, our bodies have highly developed systems of antioxidants that try to keep atoms of oxygen traveling in the right direction—into the Krebs cycle—and prevent them from making trouble elsewhere in the body.

Some of the body's major antioxidant systems include glutathione peroxidase, superoxide dismutase, catalase, and cytochrome P450. Some of these substances and the biochemical pathways they define are meant to keep oxygen heading in the right direction while others aim to keep it from heading off in the wrong direction.

Here's an analogy that might help put the two faces of oxygen—the positive face of oxygenation that feeds our cells and the negative face of oxidation that stresses them—into context:

The U.S. navy has a fleet of nuclear submarines. These remarkable ships are capable of remaining submerged in the ocean for months at a time as they travel around the world. The energy needed to power these huge machines comes from compact nuclear reactors that tap the energy of atomic nuclei to generate heat. In addition to driving the sub, this heat is used for everything on board—from scrubbing and recharging the air that the seamen breathe and purifying the water they drink to running the radar and information systems that keep them in touch and on track. If the nuclear generator on board were to fail, the lives of the crew would be imperiled.

On the other hand, the nuclear fuel needs to stay deep within the core of the reactor. Even though it produces the life-giving energy that every person on board depends on, the fuel itself is toxic. A few moments of direct exposure would create a lethal dose of radiation poisoning. The nuclear fuel must be kept within very specific "lanes" —in this case, the physical shielding of the reactor core. It's the same with oxygen. It gives us life, but only when it is directed to and kept within the "core" of the biochemical processes that use oxygen to make energy. Just like nuclear fuel escaping from the core, oxygen that escapes from the bounds of our antioxidant systems becomes very, very dangerous.

The perils of oxidative stress

When oxygen slips outside of the lanes created in the body by antioxidants, it strips electrons from nearby substances, creating positively charged ions called free radicals. As I've described, one free radical, in an effort to find an electron to rebalance itself, damages another molecule, converting it into a free radical, and so forth. This domino-like series of damaging events is known as an oxidative stress cascade.

Oxidative damage causes many problems. First off, through the cascade process, oxygen can break down essential substances in the body, degrading them and even turning them into toxins and wastes that must be removed from the body, rather than helpful substances that serve it.

Secondly, by locking up electrons, oxidatively damaged free radicals reduce the flow of electrons the body uses to create and direct energy at a cellular level. In traditional Chinese medicine, the term *ch'i* (or *qi*) is used to refer to vital energy. In biochemical terms, ch'i may be understood in terms of this flow. When the body enters a highly oxidized state, electron flow—and therefore vital energy—is reduced. We may experience this as a loss of physical energy, depression, anxiety, or other nervous system disorders, poor digestion, and a wide range of metabolic complaints ranging from constipation to diabetes. It may also manifest as weakened immunity, leading to increased susceptibility to infections or slower healing and recovery.

Finally, the presence of free radicals in the body is a trigger for many inflammatory processes. Free radicals trigger the production of NF-κB (nuclear transcription factor kappa-B), which in turn signals the production of inflammatory cytokines—immune system substances produced by the body to fight cancer and other infections. While this can be helpful if triggered at the right time, when we are constantly exposed to oxidatively damaged free radicals, the overexpression of NF-κB and its related, downstream cytokines can produce chronic inflammatory problems, including arthritic symptoms, fibromyalgia, and even cardiovascular diseases.

How our cells use oxygen

With every inhalation—each breath of air we take—oxygen is drawn down into the lungs through a branching network of finer and finer tubes called bronchi. At the end of these bronchi, the air inflates a spongy mass composed of billions of microscopic balloons called alveoli. Each alveolar bubble is wrapped in a network of tiny blood vessels so thin that the oxygen inside the alveoli passes directly into the blood. This oxygen-rich blood is then returned to the heart where it is pumped to all of the cells of the body.

Our cells, in turn, have the ability to absorb oxygen from the blood. One of the central biochemical processes within our cells takes this oxygen and delivers it, along with other nutrients, including sugars and fats, to the energy-producing centers within the cell—specialized capsules called mitochondria. Mitochondria use these nutrients as fuel to produce a molecule called adenosine triphosphate, more commonly referred to as ATP. ATP is the body's universal currency for storing and delivering energy where it's needed, for everything from running to catch a bus to processing the electrical signals in the nervous system that give rise to thought and awareness.

The Health Benefits of Xanthones

Research reveals that the xanthones from mangosteen fruit hulls exhibit antibacterial, antifungal, and anti-inflammatory properties in the laboratory—in cell cultures and animal studies. *To date, there are no published studies describing research involving human subjects.*

Investigators in Thailand found that xanthones isolated from the fruit hulls and the edible arils and seeds of mangosteen had powerful antituberculosis actions. Alpha- and beta-mangostins and garcinone B exhibited strong inhibitory effects against *Mycobacterium tuberculosis*, the bacteria that causes tuberculosis.

Researchers in India reported that several xanthones isolated from the fruit hulls of mangosteen demonstrated good inhibitory action against three fungi—*Fusarium oxysporum vasinfectum, Alternaria tenuis,* and *Dreschlera oryzae.*

Investigators in Japan found that alpha-mangostin isolated from the stem bark of *Garcinia mangostana* L. was effective against antibiotic-resistant strains of bacteria—against Vancomycin-resistant Enterococci (gram-positive cocci that cause urinary tract infections, bacteremia, bacterial endocarditis, diverticulitis, and meningitis) and methicillin-resistant *Staphylococcus aureus*, a gram-positive cocci that can cause illnesses ranging from minor skin infections to life-threatening diseases such as pneumonia, meningitis, endocarditis, toxic shock syndrome, and septicemia (a disease caused by the spread of bacteria and their toxins in the bloodstream). The investigators also observed partial synergism—the capacity to work better together than separately—between alpha-mangostin and commercially available prescription antibiotics such as ampicillin and minocycline. They opined that their findings suggested that alpha-mangostin alone or in combination with antibiotics might be useful in controlling infections.

In Thailand, many plant species have been widely used to cure infections. In 2005, researchers tested nine medicinal plant extracts to assess their activity against methicillin-resistant *Staphylococcus aureus*. They found that mangosteen extract possessed significant activity against the bacteria and attributed this activity to the presence of metabolic toxins or broad-spectrum antibacterial compounds.

They felt that the antibacterial action observed might in part be caused by the high levels of tannins in the extract, which are known to exert antimicrobial effects.

There is considerable evidence that xanthones act to reduce the synthesis of prostaglandins—potent hormone-like substances that participate in a wide range of body functions such as the contraction and relaxation of smooth muscle, the dilation and constriction of blood vessels, control of blood pressure, and the modulation of inflammation. Xanthones also prevent oxidative damage by functioning as free-radical scavengers, act as histamine and serotonin receptor blockers, and inhibit HIV-1 protease, which means they serve to inhibit viral production and reduce viral spread.

Anti-inflammatory action

Before we consider the anti-inflammatory properties of mangosteen, it's important to understand a little about the actual mechanical process of inflammation and its role in health and illness. Inflammation is a fundamental way in which the body defends itself—it's a normal, healthy, and desirable protective response to injury or irritation, even though it often produces undesirable symptoms—pain, swelling, redness, heat, and even loss of function.

Broadly speaking, inflammation is a process that occurs when the body's immune system responds to either an injury or a microbial invader (virus, bacteria, or fungi). The immune system response involves sending a variety of cells and natural chemicals to the area in question to destroy the invading microbes and repair the damage. It causes blood vessels in the area to leak, which produces swelling, and the inflamed area becomes tender and red-hot to the touch.

Let's take a closer look at what happens in an inflammatory reaction. First off, fluid containing many important proteins such as fibrin and immunoglobulins (antibodies) rushes to the site of injury, infection, or irritation. Blood vessels dilate upstream of an infection, which produces the characteristic redness and heat at the site, and they constrict just below the site. At the same time, the permeability of the capillaries, the smallest blood vessels, increases. This circulatory process causes a loss of blood plasma in the tissue, resulting in swelling, which in turn expands the tissues, putting pressure on nerves and producing pain.

At the same time, at the cellular level, white blood cells, called leukocytes, swarm around the inflamed tissue. They are mobilized to serve as phagocytes, surrounding, engulfing, and helping to eliminate bacteria and cellular debris. In the case of infection, they also assist by erecting a cellular wall at the site of the infection to prevent its spread.

Neutrophils, the most abundant form of white blood cells, are the first white blood cells to congregate in the affected area, and they are easily identified in newly inflamed tissue viewed under a microscope. They perform many vital functions, including phagocytosis and the release of extracellular chemical messengers. Neutrophils only live for a couple days, so if the inflammation persists they are gradually replaced by longer-lived white blood cells called monocytes.

When inflammation of the affected site continues over time, an entire flotilla of cells is mobilized to the scene. Along with neutrophils and monocytes, other white blood cells—including activated T-helper cells (which activate and direct other immune cells), T-cytotoxic cells (which can kill infected cells), and memory T and B cells (which recognize a specific antigen and proliferate to form antibody-producing plasma cells—quickly move to the injured or infected site.

Long-term, chronic inflammation can harm the very tissues it is meant to protect and heal. Its potential for destruction has long been evident in diseases like rheumatoid arthritis, in which inflammation damages the joints, and multiple sclerosis, in which it destroys the insulation surrounding nerve fibers. Today, scientists are coming to realize that chronic inflammation is problematical not only because it produces discomfort but also because it predisposes sufferers to many other common chronic diseases associated with aging, including atherosclerosis, diabetes, Alzheimer's disease, and osteoporosis.

Inflammation is also implicated in asthma, cirrhosis of the liver, some bowel disorders, psoriasis, meningitis, cystic fibrosis, and even cancer. The cells involved in inflammation are detected in a variety of common cancers, together with the inflammatory cytokines—proteins produced by white blood cells that act as chemical messengers between cells and can stimulate or inhibit the growth and activity of various immune cells—and the molecules that bind cytokines.

Heightened understanding and appreciation of the role of inflammation in health and illness has prompted scientists to develop new hypotheses about disease causation. For example, over time, a new model of how heart disease develops has emerged. Rather than assuming that plaque simply builds up and clogs arteries, the new model posits that immune-system cells that cause inflammation tunnel into arterial walls and engulf droplets of fat. The fat-filled cells form a plaque and inflammation thins its fibrous cap. Eventually, the cap ruptures, and the plaque's contents spill into the bloodstream, along with pro-inflammatory cytokines, which promote clotting. Without warning, the artery fills with rapidly coagulating blood cells that can form a clot that partially or completely occludes the artery and causes a heart attack or stroke.

This model suggests that preventing and reducing inflammation is key to preventing many types of heart disease. To measure inflammatory activity, doctors measure a blood marker of inflammatory activity called C-reactive protein. There is definitive evidence from multiple epidemiological (population) studies that elevated C-reactive protein is directly related to increased risk of cardiovascular disease—heart attack or stroke.

One unresolved question that continues to plague researchers is, "What causes the inflammation?" Some scientists think that oxidized fat droplets irritate the artery walls; others believe that viruses or bacteria trigger the inflammation. The pathogens (disease-causing agents) that may be involved include herpes simplex 1, a virus that causes cold sores; cytomegalovirus, which typically produces no symptoms; the bacteria involved in gum disease; *H. pylori*, which causes stomach ulcers; and *Chlamydia pneumoniae*, which causes bronchitis and pneumonia. Investigators have identified *Chlamydia* in many arterial plaques.

Inflammation probably also contributes to the development of diabetes. Elevated C-reactive protein is associated with an increased risk of developing type 2 diabetes—the most common form of diabetes. Nearly 95 percent of diabetics have type 2 diabetes. People with type 2 diabetes produce insulin, but either do not make enough insulin or their bodies do not use the insulin they make effectively. Most people who have this type of diabetes are overweight or obese.

In people with the tendency to develop diabetes and those who already suffer from it, excess body fat may contribute to inflammation. Fat cells produce cytokines, the proteins that promote inflammation, and the more fat cells that are present, the more cytokines will be produced. Research has demonstrated that people who develop type 2 diabetes tend to have higher than average levels of these cytokines. One hypothesis is that cytokines induce insulin resistance, setting the stage for diabetes.

Osteoporosis is a decrease in bone mass and bone density that places people at increased risk of fracture. Researchers believe that inflammation may play a role in the development and progress of this disease because in osteoporosis, cytokines appear to accelerate the rate at which bone is broken down. The disease often develops in women after menopause, when estrogen levels drop. Scientists believe that estrogen protects against bone loss by decreasing the production of cytokines. At menopause, when estrogen declines, cytokine levels rise, and bone mass and density diminish.

In Alzheimer's disease, inflammation occurs in and around the protein deposits—known as amyloid plaques—that accumulate in the brain. For many years, physicians thought that the plaques caused this inflammation, but researchers have found that cytokines not only promote inflammation but also are involved in creating the plaques. It also is possible that inflammation damage to nerve cells, called neurons, is implicated in the genesis of Alzheimer's disease.

Recently, investigators in Thailand looked at the neuroprotective (providing protection to nerves or any part of the body's nervous system) effects of various extracts from the fruit hull of mangosteen. They assessed the extracts based on their free-radical scavenging activity and concluded that they were potent neuroprotectants.

Asthma has long been acknowledged as an inflammatory disease, and people with asthma are often prescribed anti-inflammatory steroids to help prevent the frequency and severity of asthma attacks. Like Alzheimer's disease, osteoporosis, and diabetes, the precise mechanism of how inflammation promotes asthma has not yet been elucidated.

Inflammation plays a pivotal role in cancer. Tumors metastasize (spread) by hijacking the body's inflammatory mechanisms. Cancer cells invade neighboring tissue in much the same way that inflammatory cells invade the lining of arteries. Inflammation is also involved in angiogenesis, the growth of small blood vessels that support tumors by delivering blood supplies to them.

Laboratory and animal studies conducted in Japan have confirmed the anti-inflammatory action of xanthones. Gamma-mangostin inhibited the activities of both COX-1 and COX-2—the cyclooxygenase enzymes that control the production of prostaglandins, the potent hormone-like substances that are involved in blood pressure regulation, contraction of smooth muscle, and the mediation of pain and inflammation.

Inhibition of COX enzymes is the method of action of well-known over-the-counter pain relievers such as aspirin and ibuprofen and prescription drugs such as ketoprofen and Celebrex. Although these drugs do reduce inflammation, their frequent unpleasant side effects, including gastrointestinal ulcers and bleeding, have prompted research for equally effective alternatives with fewer or no side effects.

Many scientists are excited about the prospect of harnessing and concentrating mangosteen's anti-inflammatory properties in much the same way that willow bark's (Salix) have been. Historically, willow bark was used as an anti-inflammatory, which later resulted in isolation of the pure compound salicylic acid, and its acetylated (the addition of an acetyl group—acetic acid, CH_3CO-) derivative acetylsalicylate, better known as aspirin.

Along with their role in inflammation, COX-2 enzymes have been found to have a role in tumor development. Many different types of cancer, including lung, colon, and breast cancer, have been found to have high tissue levels of COX-2. Researchers believe that COX-2 is involved in a range of actions related to tumor growth, serving to limit apoptosis (programmed cell death) and increase cell proliferation, promoting angiogenesis and increasing the invasiveness of malignant cells. Naturally occurring COX-2 inhibitors may be able to exert preventive and therapeutic anticancer effects. Substances that inhibit COX enzymes are important in the search for new anti-inflammatory and anticancer agents, and nature is a valuable resource for identifying molecules with these actions.

Xanthones may help to prevent and treat cancer

Other research has found that six xanthones from the pericarps of mangosteen, including alpha-mangostin, inhibited growth of human leukemia cells. Some scientists hypothesize that alpha-mangostin mediates a mitochondrial pathway in apoptosis by causing cells to swell, lose their membrane potential, and decrease their intracellular energy. The investigators concluded that, "alpha-mangostin and its analogs would be candidates for preventive and therapeutic application for cancer treatment."

A xanthone called garcinone E exerts cytotoxic effects against human hepatocellular carcinoma (liver cancer) cells, and extract from mangosteen rind was found to have potent antiproliferative, antioxidative, and apoptotic effects against human breast cancer cells. The researchers in Thailand who reported the anticancer action of xanthones against human breast cancer suggested that this antioxidant compound has the potential to prevent cancer as well as to treat it.

In the spring of 2006, researchers at The Ohio State University published the results of their studies of mangosteen and its cancer prevention properties. Using chromatography of an extract of the pericarp, they isolated two new xanthones and twelve known xanthones and determined which xanthones had the strongest antioxidant action. They identified 8-hydroxycudraxanthone G, gartanin, alpha-mangostin, gamma-mangostin, and smeathxanthone A as the most active and found that alpha-mangostin had some of the strongest ability to inhibit growth of precancerous cells.

The same year, investigators in Thailand reported similar, and even more promising, results. They identified three new prenylated xanthones—mangostenones C (1), D (2), and E (3)—and tested their anticancer effects along with sixteen known xanthones isolated from the young (seven-week-old) fruit of *Garcinia mangostana*. They observed cytotoxic properties against three human cancer cell lines, epidermoid carcinoma of the mouth, breast cancer, and small cell lung cancer. Alpha-mangostin displayed the most potent effects against the breast cancer cells with anticancer activity greater than that of the anticancer drug ellipticine.

Supporting heart health

Many epidemiological studies indicate that consuming dietary poly-phenolic compounds is beneficial in the prevention of cardiovascular diseases. Xanthones and xanthone derivatives have been shown to have beneficial effects on some cardiovascular diseases, including ischemic heart disease—problems caused by a decreased blood supply due to narrowing of the coronary arteries; atherosclerosis—clogging, narrowing, and hardening of the large arteries and medium-sized blood vessels that can lead to stroke, heart attack, eye problems, and kidney problems; hypertension (high blood pressure); and thrombosis (formation of blood clots in veins deep inside the legs).

The protective effects of xanthones for the cardiovascular system may in part be attributed to their antioxidant and anti-inflammatory action, however they also inhibit platelet aggregation—instances when platelets arrive at, and stick to, the site of injury in a blood vessel. In terms of heart health, platelets aggregate at the site of plaque formations along blood vessel walls, which leads to the development of localized blood clots, which further block the flow of blood in the artery. Xanthones also exert antithrombotic actions—preventing or interfering with the formation of thrombi (fibrinous clots formed in a blood vessel or in a chamber of the heart)—and vasorelaxant activities, which increase blood flow. Another possible explanation of xanthones' observed ability to prevent and reduce atherosclerosis is that they oppose endogenous nitric oxide synthase inhibitors. This means that they limit the amount of nitric oxide, which is proinflammatory, produced by the body.

Mangosteen may also support heart health by helping to reduce and normalize blood cholesterol levels. Investigators in Australia and Thailand posited that because mangosteen inhibits oxidative (free radical) damage, then it might serve to reduce the oxidation of "bad" LDL cholesterol in the blood. The investigators found that the xanthones from mangosteen effectively inhibit LDL oxidation.

A Ripe and Possibly Royal History

One of the earliest reports of mangosteen trees was in a 1770 dispatch from Captain Cook. Writing from Java, he raved about the fruit, ". . . they are about the size of a crab apple, of deep yellow brown color when mature . . . when they are eaten . . . nothing can be more delicious, a happy mixture of the tart and the sweet."

The first introduction of mangosteen in the United Kingdom is credited to Anton Pantaleon Hove. Hove was dispatched by Sir Joseph Banks, head of the Royal Botanical Gardens at Kew and president of the Royal Society, to seek better strains of cottonseeds from India. Along with the seeds, he returned with mangosteen plants that arrived safely in Plymouth, England, in 1789.

The first recorded fruiting of mangosteen trees in the United Kingdom took place in 1855. Since fruiting mangosteen is no small feat, this accomplishment, by the gardener at the ancestral home of the Dukes of Northumberland, was duly noted in great detail. Apparently, a greenhouse complex was heated to maintain a steady tropical temperature to offset the temperate British climate. The seeds were obtained, so the article goes, by a Captain White from Calcutta and grown in large tubs.

Flowers formed on one or both of the two trees in November of 1854. One tree was described as about 15 feet high and 9 feet wide. The Royal Horticultural Society acknowledged the magnitude of this accomplishment and the fruit received the Gold Banksian Medal, the first time such an honor was bestowed upon a single fruit.

By 1855, mangosteen trees were growing and fruiting in greenhouses in several parts of England. The plants were also introduced to the New World, including the Caribbean. By 1880, mangosteen trees were established in the public gardens of Jamaica as well as on Trinidad and Dominica.

A Ripe and Possibly Royal History (continued)

Many marketers of mangosteen juice and extract repeat the adage that Queen Victoria tasted the mangosteen, loved it and declared it her favorite fruit. Although some historians claim that Queen Victoria was in attendance when the fruit was first presented in the United Kingdom, there is no proof that confirms this contention. Others have observed that had the Queen been present, it would have been sufficiently newsworthy that the press would most certainly have documented it, and no such documentation has been found.

The Royal Archives contains a letter dated May 5, 1855, from Eleanor, the Duchess of Northumberland, addressed to Queen Victoria requesting permission to send a mangosteen fruit to her Majesty. This letter calls into question the claim that the Queen had already seen the fruit and there is no documented evidence that the Queen subsequently received the fruit or ever tasted the mangosteen.

Similarly, despite many references describing the Queen's willingness to reward the first person to bring her a fresh mangosteen, there is no evidence that Queen Victoria ever offered any reward in exchange for a fresh mangosteen. It is also improbable that Queen Victoria had any role in dubbing mangosteen the queen of tropical fruit. More likely this expression is a translation of an old Thai or Malay description of mangosteen.

Growing Mangosteen

The mangosteen tree is a slow-growing tropical pyramidal evergreen that grows as tall as 25 meters in warm, wet, tropical climates—temperatures below 40 degrees Fahrenheit freeze and kill these sensitive, exotic plants, and they cannot tolerate temperatures above 100 degrees. The young seedlings are even more fragile, perishing if the temperature drops to 45 degrees Fahrenheit. Seedlings and mature trees must be sheltered from high winds and salt spray.

Mangosteen most likely originated in Southeast Asia, possible in the Sunda Islands and the Moluccas in the western part of the Malay Archipelago. Today it grows in Northern Australia, Brazil, Burma, Central America, Hawaii, Southern India, Indonesia, Malaysia, Sri Lanka, Thailand, Vietnam, and other tropical countries. Mangosteen thrives in warm humid environments and deep, rich, organic soil, especially sandy loam or laterite—a clay that is high in iron and aluminum.

Mangosteen is only found as a cultivated female tree—male trees are virtually nonexistent. It is likely a hybrid between two species (*G. malaccensis* and *G. hombroniana*) and is structurally and functionally an intermediate between these two species. Some scientists have hypothesized that all mangosteen trees originated from a single clone. Mangosteen plants reproduce asexually in a process known as parthenogenesis—the production of living organisms from seeds. Because mangosteen is exceedingly difficult to propagate using plant cuttings and stems, most trees are produced from seeds, which remain viable for just a few days.

Young plants grow from five to fifteen years and develop dark brown or black flaky bark. Mangosteen trees flower annually or twice a year following particularly dry spells. Some of the most fruitful mangosteen trees grow on the banks of streams, lakes, ponds, or canals where the roots are almost always wet. A period of dry weather just before blooming time and during flowering yields abundant hermaphrodite flowers and fruit. The flowers are yellow-green with thick, red-tinged petals. They may produce fruit as early as seven years after planting, but most trees don't bear fruit until they're at least ten years old and some do not produce fruit until they are twenty years old.

The first harvest of fruit may number from two to three hundred, and the average yield of a full-grown tree is about five hundred fruits. The crop yield steadily increases up to the thirtieth year of bearing when one to two thousand fruits may be harvested from a single tree. Trees between the ages of twenty and forty-five years have been known to produce two to three thousand fruits! After this peak, productivity gradually declines but the mangosteen tree continues to bear fruit until it's one hundred years old.

Mangosteen fruits are fully ripe 119 days after flowering but fruit may be harvested as early as 113 days. The mangosteen is usually hand-picked to prevent damage to the pericarp. Placed in dry, warm containers, unripe mangosteens may be stored for about three weeks. When they are stored for prolonged periods, their outer skins toughen, the rinds become rubbery, and ultimately, the rinds harden and become difficult to open and the flesh dries out. Ripe mangosteens will keep well for about four weeks in cool storage, but with optimal storage conditions—temperatures of 39 to 42 degrees Fahrenheit and a relatively high humidity of 85 to 90 percent—they can last as long as forty-nine days.

Today, the major growers and producers of mangosteen are Thailand, Malaysia, Indonesia, and the Philippines. Despite tremendous demand in local and export markets, the area devoted to cultivating mangosteen is relatively small and production is currently insufficient to meet market demands.

The main fruiting season varies depending on where mangosteen is grown. In Thailand, it is harvested from May through July; in peninsular Malaysia, the fruiting season runs from June through August; in the Philippines, the season spans from July to September; and in eastern Malaysia, fruiting occurs from November through January.

Savoring Mangosteen

Fresh mangosteens are rare and delicious treats. Since they don't ripen further once they have been harvested, choose fruits that have no skin imperfections or major discoloration. Bright green stems indicate fresh, quality fruit. The choicest fruit is not hard and yields when pressed gently. Mangosteens will keep for a few days without refrigeration and cool storage extends their shelf life. Refrigeration can cause cold damage, and freezing compromises both the flavor and texture of the fruit. Should you choose to refrigerate fresh mangosteen, wrap it in newspaper and store it in the upper part of the refrigerator.

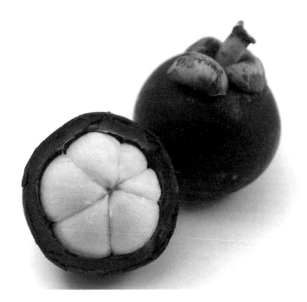

In terms of flavor, scent, and texture, mangosteens are best eaten fresh. Eat them out of hand or add them to tropical fruit salads. To open the fruit, the simplest method is to place it in the palm of your hand with the stem on top, and use your fingers to exert gentle pressure on the upper half until the shell opens. Another option is to cut through the diameter of the shell all the way around, and then simply lift off the top and spoon out the flesh of the fruit.

Mangosteen is also available frozen or canned in syrup. As the nutrition facts reveal, like most fruits, mangosteen is low in sodium and fat, contains no cholesterol, and a one-cup serving of canned fruit contains 143 calories.

Sadly, many of the nutritional benefits of mangosteen are not in its sweet pulp but in the tough, bitter rind. For this reason, people seeking the nutritional benefits of xanthones often prefer juice, dried fruit, powders, extracts, and other preparations that contain the key nutrients found in mangosteen pericarp. Another benefit of these mangosteen preparations is that many do not contain the high concentrations of natural sugar found in the fresh fruit.

Mangosteen Goes Mainstream

From its traditional uses in native tropical cultures around the world to groundbreaking research in modern biomedical laboratories, mangosteen is clearly entering the mainstream of American cuisine, culture, and complementary, integrative, and alternative medicine and healing. One day soon, mangosteen may become as well known as the more traditional tropical fruits such as mango, papaya, pineapple, guava, and kiwi.

Nutrition Facts

Serving Size 1 cup, drained 196g (196g)

Amount Per Serving

Calories 143   Calories from Fat 10

% Daily Value*

Total Fat 1g	2%
Saturated Fat	0%
Trans Fat	
Cholesterol 0mg	0%
Sodium 14mg	1%
Total Carbohydrate 35g	12%
Dietary Fiber 4g	14%
Sugars	
Protein 1g	

Vitamin A	1%	• Vitamin C	9%
Calcium	2%	• Iron	3%

*Percent Daily Values are based on a 2,000 calorie diet. Your daily values may be higher or lower depending on your calorie needs:

		Calories	2,000	2,500
Total Fat	Less than		65g	80g
Sat Fat	Less than		20g	25g
Cholesterol	Less than		300mg	300mg
Sodium	Less than		2,400mg	2,400mg
Total Carbohydrate			300g	375g
Fiber			25g	30g

Calories per gram:
Fat 9   •   Carbohydrate 4   •   Protein 4

NutritionData.com

References

Chairungsrilerd N., et al. "Histaminergic and serotonergic receptor blocking substances from the medicinal plant *Garcinia mangostana.*" *Planta Med* 1996; 62 (5): 471–72.

Chen S.X., Wan M., Loh B.N. "Active constituents against HIV-1 protease from *Garcinia mangostana.*" *Planta Med* 1996; 62 (4): 381–82.

dela Cruz F.S. "Status report on genetic resources of mangosteen (*Garcinia mangostana* L.) in Southeast Asia." International Plant Genetic Resource Institute, Malaysia, 2001.

Gopalakrishnan G., Banumathi B., Suresh G. "Evaluation of the antifungal activity of natural xanthones from *Garcinia mangostana* and their synthetic derivatives." *J Nat Prod* 1997; 60 (5): 519–24.

Ho C.K., Huang Y.L., Chen C.C. "Garcinone E, a xanthone derivative, has potent cytotoxic effect against hepatocellular carcinoma cell lines." *Planta Med* 2002; 68 (11): 975–79.

International Centre for Underutilized Crops. Fruits for the Future. Factsheet No. 8, United Kingdom Department for International Development Forestry Research Programme, 2003.

Jiang D.J., Dai Z., Li Y.J. "Pharmacological effects of xanthones as cardiovascular protective agents." *Cardiovasc Drug Rev* 2004; 22 (2): 91–102.

Jung H.A., et al. "Antioxidant xanthones from the pericarp of *Garcinia mangostana* (Mangosteen)." *J Agric Food Chem* 2006; 54 (6): 2077–82.

Matsumoto K., et al. "Induction of apoptosis by xanthones from mangosteen in human leukemia cell lines." *J Nat Prod* 2003; 66 (8): 1124–27.

Matsumoto K., et al. "Preferential target is mitochondria in alpha-mangostin-induced apoptosis in human leukemia HL60 cells." *Bioorg Med Chem* 2004; 12(22): 5799–806.

Moongkarndi P., et al. "Antiproliferation, antioxidation and induction of apoptosis by *Garcinia mangostana* (mangosteen) on SKBR3 human breast cancer cell line." *J Ethnopharmacol* 2004; 90 (1): 161–66.

Morton, J. F. *Fruits of warm climates*. Florida Flair Books. 1987: 310–14.

Nakatani K., et al. "Inhibition of cyclooxygenase and prostaglandin E2 synthesis by gamma-mangostin, a xanthone derivative in mangosteen, in C6 rat glioma cells." *Biochem Pharmacol* 2002; 63 (1): 73–79.

Sakagami Y., et al. "Antibacterial activity of alpha-mangostin against vancomycin resistant Enterococci (VRE) and synergism with antibiotics." *Phytomedicine* . 2005 Mar;12 (3): 203–08.

Suksamrarn S., et al. "Antimycobacterial activity of prenylated xanthones from the fruits of *Garcinia mangostana*." *Chem Pharm Bull* (Tokyo) 2003; 51(7): 857–59.

Suksamrarn S., et al. "Cytotoxic prenylated xanthones from the young fruit of *Garcinia mangostana*." *Chem Pharm Bull* (Tokyo) 2006 Mar; 54 (3): 301–05.

Voravuthikunchai S.P., Kitpipit L. "Activity of medicinal plant extracts against hospital isolates of methicillin-resistant *Staphylococcus aureus*." *Clin Microbiol and Infection* 2005; 11 (6): 510–12.

Weecharangsan W., et al. "Antioxidative and neuroprotective activities of extracts from the fruit hull of mangosteen (*Garcinia mangostana* Linn.)." *Med Princ Pract* 2006; 15 (4): 281–87.

About the Author

Barbara Wexler is a medical writer and chronic disease epidemiologist who brings more than twenty-five years of experience as a clinician, researcher, educator, and administrator to the articles and texts she prepares for professional and consumer audiences. A graduate of Sarah Lawrence College and the Yale University College of Medicine, School of Epidemiology and Public Health, Wexler is interested in evidence-based complementary and integrative medicine.